Introduction

I want to thank you and congratulate you for purchasing the book, *"Dukan Diet Recipes – 42 Delicious Dukan Diet Recipes For Weight Loss"*.

Are you tired of trying different diets to lose weight but are unsuccessful? Do you want a diet that will be easy to follow? If this is you, then the Dukan Diet is the perfect diet for you. While most diets may be monotonous, restrictive and even boring, the Dukan Diet is interesting and easy to follow without it being too restrictive.

This book explains what the Dukan Diet is and the different phases of the Dukan Diet. You will also have over forty recipes that you can try at home in your journey to lose weight.

Thanks again for purchasing this book, I hope you enjoy it!

Sara Banks

What Is The Dukan Diet?

With there being so many diets being developed each day, you may wonder whether there is any specific diet that will best help you to lose weight. While some diets may require you to only take fluids within a certain period and others requiring you to fast several days, you can be overwhelmed with all the restrictions. However, who said losing weight has to be too restrictive. It is still possible to eat the foods you love but in moderation.

The Dukan diet is simply a lifestyle meal plan designed to help you lose weight in a quick and healthy way. This diet usually comprises of high proteins, low carbs and moderate fats. Since the diet is low in carbohydrates, your body is forced to start burning fats when it does not get enough carbohydrates for energy.

There are four phases of the Dukan Diet namely the attack phase, the cruise phase, the consolidation phase, and the stabilization phase.

The Attack Phase

The attack phase is largely intake of protein for up to seven days. As such, you will mostly encounter fat free dairy products, lean meats, tofu, seitan and eggs with little carbohydrates but with adequate fats.

The Cruise Phase

The cruise phase on the other hand incorporates non-starchy veggies with proteins, with at least thirty minutes of exercise every day, and two tablespoons of oat bran.

The Consolidation Phase

This phase is a little longer than the second phase, and has one protein day during the week, with all the others blended in a mixture of proteins, carbohydrates, and some fruits except grapes, bananas, dried fruits or cherries. You may add some carbohydrates in the consolidation phase once you have lost some pounds.

The Stabilization Phase

The stabilization phase is basically a guideline for what you are supposed to eat and do for the rest of your life. You can decide to make Thursdays your all protein day, take three teaspoons of oat bran every day, and avoid escalators or elevators.

Sticking to the Dukan diet can help you lose weight fast and avoid certain diseases associated with being overweight and obese. Such diseases include hypertension, diabetes and heart attack. In addition, this diet helps you lose significant weight in a short time, which gives you more confidence to follow through. Moreover, it is a lifelong program that is very easy to follow.

Attack Phase Recipes

1. Chilli And Ginger Roast Chicken

Ingredients

1 lemon

1 whole medium-sized chicken

1 cube of fresh ginger

1 red chilli pepper

1 teaspoon of paprika

3 cloves of garlic

2 teaspoons of dried oregano

Instructions

Pre-heat the oven to 190 degrees C or 200 if your oven does not have a fan.

Cut lemon into two halves, dent the lemon, squeeze some of the juice into the cavity of the chicken, and press the lemon halves inside. Find a roasting tin to put the chicken.

Remove the green stalk and ends of the red chilli, slice it at the middle and remove the seeds. Cut into small pieces and put into the roasting tin with the chicken breast.

Peel and cut the ginger into small equal pieces.

Divide each of the 3 garlic cloves along their length.

Stab the chicken breast with a sharp knife to make room for the ginger, garlic and chilli.

Sprinkle the oregano and paprika on the top.

Place in the oven for 1 ½ to 2 hours to cook until the chicken is set and turns brown.

Once cooked, remove the chicken and cut it; ensure that that there is no blood and the juices are clear and then serve.

2. Lemon Chicken Skewers

Ingredients

For the marinade:

1 chopped red chilli

Juice of one lemon

1 cube of fresh sliced ginger

1 Large sliced clove of garlic

A handful of fresh chopped coriander

For the dip:

2 tablespoons of chopped fresh parsley

250g of fat free Greek yogurt

½ teaspoon of paprika

2 tablespoons of chopped fresh chives

Salt and pepper

Instructions

Mix all the marinade ingredients in a bowl.

Chop the chicken breasts into chunks. Add them to the marinade, stir to mix well, and then cover with cling film. Put in the fridge to marinate for at least half an hour. You can leave it for an hour or more for best results if you have the time.

Prepare the dip by mixing all the ingredients in a small bowl, add a pinch of salt and pepper to taste, and then refrigerate while the chicken is marinating.

Cook in the oven under medium grill for about twenty-five minutes until it turns golden brown.

Serve with the parsley dip and dill.

3. Caraway Flavored Pork Chops

Ingredients

2 pork chops

1 tablespoon of caraway seeds

1 lemon

Salt and pepper to taste

Instructions

Heat the oven to 180 degrees C. Remove any visible fats from the pork chops using a chopping board and put on a plate.

Crush the caraway seeds into powder using a pestle and mortar then sprinkle around the pork chops then add salt and pepper to taste.

Sauté the meat using a slightly greased non-stick pan under medium heat. Put the pork chops in a roasting tin once they are set and have turned brown. Let it cook and squeeze the lemon juice around the pork chops and serve.

4. Thai Chicken Patties

Ingredients

For the chicken patties:

1 chopped garlic clove

1 small, peeled and chopped piece of fresh ginger

350g of ground chicken

4 tablespoons of fresh coriander

1 green, roughly chopped chilli

½ red onion chopped

For the dip:

2 tablespoons of chopped fresh chives

250g of 0% fat Greek yogurt

A splash of lemon juice

3 chopped spring onions

Salt and black pepper to taste

Instructions

Prepare the dip by mixing all the ingredients in a food processor or blender, add salt and pepper to taste and puree until smooth. Pour into a small bowl, and use a cling film to cover. Put in the fridge while you prepare the chicken patties.

Put all the Thai patties ingredients except the chicken in a food processor and blend. Pour these ingredients into the chicken and mix thoroughly. Mould six small cakes using your hand.

Cook the patties in a lightly greased non-stick pan under medium heat until they turn golden brown. This can take ten minutes.

Serve with the Greek yogurt dip.

5. Steak Pizzaiola

Ingredients

2 lean beef frying steaks or veal escalopes

2 sliced cloves of garlic

2 tablespoons of tomato paste

Cooking spray to grease the pan

A handful of chopped flat leaf parsley

Black pepper to taste

Instructions

Dilute the tomato paste with a few tablespoons of warm water in a small bowl then grease the frying pan with the cooking spray and put the veal escalopes, without the hob, in the pan.

Daub the tomato paste around the meat, and then add garlic to top, with half of the chopped parsley. Let this cook for around fifteen minutes over medium heat or until they are properly cooked.

Add some hot water if the tomato sauce gets too thick while cooking. Add freshly ground black pepper when the steaks are done, and then sprinkle with the rest of the chopped parsley and serve when hot.

6. Spanish sea food

Ingredients

A few drops of extra-virgin olive oil

1 packet of refrigerated and pre-cooked seafood mix (prawns, mussels, squid)

1 teaspoon of tomato puree

1 clove of finely chopped or crushed garlic

Chopped chives

½ chopped red chilli

Salt and pepper to taste

Instructions

Put the extra virgin oil in a pan then let it melt under medium heat and add the garlic.

Add the seafood when the garlic has browned. Bring them to a boil then add chili, salt, and pepper to taste.

Let these cook for 5 minutes before you add the tomato puree.

Leave for another 5 minutes to cook then top with the chives and serve.

7. Tuna and tzatziki sauce

Ingredients

2 tuna steaks

For the marinade

Juice of one lime

2 tablespoons of teriyaki sauce

Black pepper to taste

For the tzatziki

1/3 of a de-seeded and roughly chopped cucumber

250g 0% fat Greek yogurt

Juice of one lime

½ clove of crushed garlic

Salt and pepper to taste

2 tablespoons of chopped fresh dill

Instructions

Mix the teriyaki sauce in a small bowl with the limejuice. Dip the tuna steaks in the bowl, and roll them until they are fully covered in the marinade. Put in the fridge to cool for at least 30 minutes but make sure to cover with cling film.

Prepare the dip before the thirty minutes are up by blending the garlic, cucumber, lemon juice and dill in a blender or food processor until a smooth mixture is formed. Pour Greek yogurt into a bowl, and then blend in with the cucumber paste. Cover with cling film and refrigerate.

Once you have marinated the chicken enough, remove from the fridge then spray a non stick pan with oil spray and place over medium heat and then add the tuna steaks. Depending on your cooking preferences, you can sear for around two minutes if you want it fairly red, or more if you want it thoroughly cooked. Be sure not to overcook it though. Remove the tzatziki dip and serve with the tuna.

8. Mini Burgers

Ingredients

1 egg

600g of lean turkey mince

1 tablespoon of Cajun spice mix

2 tablespoons of oat bran

2 small chopped cloves of garlic

1 green chilli, chopped (optional)

Instructions

Blend in the mince with the rest of the ingredients in a bowl using a fork. You can use a food processor if you have it to speed up things.

Shape the turkey mixture using your hands to get eight small burgers.

Place a griddle pan over medium heat and preheat it for about five minutes.

Arrange the burgers on the griddle pan, and let them cook until they are done and the meat is cooked.

Best served hot with 0% fat Greek yogurt.

9. Rosemary Beef burgers

Ingredients

For the burgers

1 whole egg

450g lean beef mince

2 tablespoons of chopped fresh rosemary

3tablespoons of oat bran

Freshly ground black pepper

1 teaspoon of nutmeg

For the dip:

1 teaspoon of smoked paprika

250g of 0% fat Greek yogurt

2 teaspoons of dried dill

Instructions

Blend in all the ingredients for the yogurt dip in a bowl then cover with cling film and set in the fridge to cool.

Mix the rest of the ingredients for the burgers in a food processor, or in a bowl with a fork if you do not have the processor.

Make ten burgers from the mixture by molding using your hands.

Place a griddle pan over high heat and let it heat up for about five minutes.

Place your burgers on the griddle pan then let them cook until the burgers turn brown and the meat is well cooked.

Serve hot with the dill and paprika dip.

10. Salmon baked omelet

Ingredients

200g smoked salmon

6 eggs

2 tablespoons of fat-free natural yogurt

1 tablespoon of chopped fresh chives

1 tablespoon of dried dill

Freshly ground black pepper

Instructions

Pre-heat the oven to 180 degrees C.

Chop the smoked salmon roughly then set 2/3 aside to use with the eggs, and the remaining 1/3 to top the omelet.

Mix the yogurt, dried drill and the eggs in a bowl.

Add the chopped salmon, and mix well. Add the freshly ground black pepper to season.

Pour the egg mixture into a tin mold made of silicone so that you don't use any extra fat and the omelet does not stick to the mold.

Place the remaining salmon close together at the top of the omelet, and add the chopped chives at the top.

Place in the oven for about forty minutes to cook.

Serve.

11. Turkey Kebabs

Ingredients

Juice of ½ lemon

500g of diced turkey thigh (or chicken breast)

2 teaspoons of paprika

2 cloves of crushed garlic

½ teaspoon of turmeric

½ teaspoon of ground ginger

1/3 teaspoon of saffron

½ teaspoon of black pepper

Instructions

Strip the turkey cubes of any visible fat and put them in a bowl. Add the rest of the ingredients, and blend them in using your hands to make sure that each piece of meat is covered with the spice mixture. Put this in the fridge for about one hour to marinate but be sure to cover the bowl with a cling film. The longer it stays chilled, the better the results.

Put the kebabs together using metal or bamboo skewers and place them aside.

Place a griddle pan under high heat for about five minutes before you put the kebabs. Let them cook until the meat is done and turns golden brown.

12. Salmon and Cream Cheese Wrap

Ingredients

2 whole eggs or egg whites

A few slices of smoked salmon

3 tablespoons of 0% fat Greek yogurt

1 tablespoon of low fat cream cheese

3 tablespoons of oat bran

1 chives flavored oat bran galette

Black pepper

Instructions

Mix all the ingredients in a bowl using a whisk until a smooth batter forms. Add a little yogurt if the batter comes out too thick. Add one tablespoon of chopped chives to the mixture.

Lightly grease the bottom of a non-stick pan and pour half of the batter. Place the pan over medium heat until the pancake turns golden brown on all sides. Remove and repeat this process for the second pancake.

Let the pancake stay for a couple of minutes to cool down. Press the cream cheese on the galette and top with the smoked salmon. Add black pepper to season.

Fold and seal the wraps then slice halfway and enjoy.

13. Bacon And Scrambled Eggs Sandwich

Ingredients

2 oat bran galettes

4 eggs

1 pack of turkey bacon rashers

A pinch of dried dill

4 tablespoons of skimmed milk

Salt and pepper

For the pancakes

2 whole eggs or egg whites

3 tablespoons of 0% fat Greek yogurt

3 tablespoons of oat bran

Instructions for the pancakes

Mix all the ingredients in a bowl using a whisk until a smooth batter forms. Add a little yogurt if the batter comes out too thick.

Lightly grease the bottom of a non-stick pan and pour half of the batter in. Place the pan over medium heat until the pancake turns golden brown on all sides. Remove and repeat this process for the second pancake, place on a plate and cover to keep warm.

Instructions for the scrambled eggs mix

Break 4 eggs into a bowl, and add the skimmed milk. Whisk the mixture together until the milk and eggs have blended. Add salt and pepper to taste, and then sprinkle with a pinch of dried dill. If you do not use dill, you can use any herb of your choice such as tarragon as a replacement.

Spray a non-stick pan with vegetable oil spray and place it under medium heat for a few minutes. Add the egg mixture when the pan is hot enough, allow it to cook for a couple of minutes, and then pull the eggs on the edges to the center with a spatula. Fold the eggs until they are done but moist.

Spray another non stick pan with vegetable oil spray then place it under medium heat and fry the turkey rashers. Place them on the pancakes then add the scrambled eggs at the top, and then make two sandwiches by folding the oat bran galettes.

Serve hot.

14. Oat Bran Galette With Toffee Yogurt

Ingredients

2 tablespoons of oat bran

1 egg

1 teaspoon of sweetener

2 tablespoons of 0% fat Greek yogurt

1 small pot of low fat toffee yogurt

Instructions

Start by first mixing the oat bran, egg, sweetener and yogurt until smooth.

Lightly grease a non-stick pan and place it under medium heat until hot. Pour in half of the mixture and cook the pancake on both sides until golden brown. Put this in a plate and cover to keep warm.

Do this for the second pancake. Serve this with the toffee yogurt. You can take this with any other low fat yogurt of your choice like vanilla.

15. Coffee Frappuccino

Ingredients

For the oat bran galette

2 whole eggs or egg whites

3 tablespoons of 0% fat Greek yogurt

3 tablespoons of oat bran

Your favorite herbs or spices

For the filling

2 tablespoons of low fat cream cheese

Lean cooked meat (ham, beef, chicken or turkey ham)

Instructions

Mix all the ingredients in a bowl using a whisk until a smooth batter forms. Add a little yogurt if the batter comes out too thick. Flavor with your favorite spices and/or herbs.

Lightly grease the bottom of a non-stick pan and pour half of the batter in. Place the pan over medium heat until the pancake turns golden brown on all sides. Remove and repeat this process for the second pancake, place on a plate and cover to keep warm.

Slice the galette into two and spread a layer of cream cheese on both sides like with bread. Stuff these with your cooked meat, and serve.

16. Homemade yogurt

Ingredients

1 large tub of fat-free natural yogurt

3 tablespoons of boiling water

3 teaspoons of sugar-free jelly

Instructions

Mix the sugar-free jelly powder with boiling water in a small bowl until it completely dissolves and no lumps are visible at the bottom. Leave this for two minutes to cool down.

Blend in the jelly syrup and yogurt in a food processor until they are properly mixed. Use a spoon if you do not have a food processor to mix, but make sure there are no lumps left at the bottom.

Instructions using an ice cream machine

Pour the jelly mixture and yogurt in the ice cream machine and do as the manual says. This should take less than one hour to get a smooth and gluten free yogurt.

Instructions when not using an ice cream machine

Pour your mixture into a freezer safe container then cover, and wait for thirty minutes to set.

Remove the container from the freezer after thirty minutes, or when it has set and stir thoroughly to break any ice crystals that may have formed and return it to the freezer. Do this every thirty minutes until the frozen yogurt reaches the right consistency. Serve immediately. This is a slightly longer process, and can take up to four hours before the yogurt is ready.

Cruise Phase Recipes

17. **Beef Stew**

Ingredients

2 tablespoons of corn flour

350g of lean beef strips

2 sliced medium carrots

Freshly ground black pepper

3 roughly chopped celery sticks

300g of peeled shallots

1 ½ pint of reduced sodium beef stock

8 sliced chestnut mushrooms

1 teaspoon of dried thyme

2 bay leaves

Low fat cooking spray

1 teaspoon of dried oregano

Instructions

Pre-heat the oven to 180 degrees C.

Place the beef in a bowl, coat with corn flour, and sprinkle freshly ground black pepper.

Place shallots, carrots, celery, herbs and mushrooms in a casserole dish and set aside.

Take a non-stick pan and spray it with low fat cooking spray at the bottom. Turn the heat to medium high and let the beef cook until it is browned.

When done, transfer it to the casserole dish with the vegetable and mix with beef stock.

Cover the casserole dish with a lid, place it in the oven, and let it cook for 2 hours or until the meat has cooked well and is tender and the stock becomes thick.

18. Stuffed Peppers

Ingredients

300g of lean minced beef

4 red peppers

4 tablespoons of oat bran

1 egg

1 teaspoon of paprika

2 cloves of garlic, crushed

Instructions

Pre-heat the oven to 180 degrees C.

Divide the peppers halfway across their lengths then de-seed and remove any white flesh.

Place the peppers in a greaseproof paper lined with a roasting tin and cook until they soften up. This can take about twenty minutes.

While these are cooking, prepare your stuffing by putting the egg, minced beef, 2 tablespoons of oat bran, paprika, and garlic in a food processor and mix. You can mix them in a bowl using a fork if you do not have a food processor.

Remove the peppers from the oven, drain excess water and stuff with minced meat mixture.

Sprinkle the rest of the oat bran over the peppers and return in the oven to bake for 30 minutes until the meat is done and the oat bran crust turns brown.

19. Chicken Shirataki Noodle Soup

Ingredients

One 150g pack of pre-cooked shirataki noodles

1 medium chopped carrot

Low fat cooking spray

3 chopped spring onions

3 chopped celery sticks

1 tablespoon of corn flour, melted in 2 tablespoons of cold water

1 teaspoon of fresh grated ginger

1 ½ pints of reduced salt chicken stock

1 teaspoon of all spice

1 sliced medium courgette

180g of mangetout

200g of pre-packaged or leftover cooked chicken

2 tablespoons of low sodium soy sauce

Instructions

First, prepare the noodles. Put them in a sink colander, rinse with warm water and then pour in a cooking dish with boiling water for about two minutes. Rinse and put aside.

Take a non-stick pan, spray it with low fat cooking spray at the bottom, and cook the celery, carrot, and spring onions under medium heat for about 3 minutes.

Mix in the grated ginger while stirring, and let it simmer for some thirty seconds.

Add the spice, corn flour, courgette, chicken stock, cooked chicken, mange tout, and simmer for another 15 minutes or until the stock has reduced down and all the veggies are tender and cooked.

Add the soy sauce and the shirataki noodles then simmer for 2 minutes,   and   serve!

20. Cottage Pie

Ingredients

4 carrots: 1 chopped finely for the pie filling, and 3 chopped roughly for the mash topping

½ finely chopped onion

400g lean beef mince or turkey mince

3 finely chopped celery sticks

½ teaspoon of dried thyme

2 tablespoons of tomato paste

½ teaspoon of marjoram

½ teaspoon of dried rosemary

2 teaspoons of corn flour, melted in 2 tablespoons of cold water

1 pint of reduced salt beef stock

Low fat cooking spray

1 swede, cut into chunks

Salt and pepper

Instructions

Put the swede and roughly chopped carrots in a deep pan then add boiling water and leave to simmer. Meanwhile, prepare the cottage pie filling.

Spray the bottom of a non-stick pan with low fat cooking pan then put the chopped onion and let it cook under medium heat until it turns golden brown.

Add the celery, finely chopped carrot, and 3 tablespoons of hot water. Leave it for another three minutes.

Add the tomato paste, beef mince, and herbs, and salt and pepper to taste. You may add 1 tablespoon of Italian herb mix if you like. Cook for ten minutes or until the meat is almost set.

Add beef stock topping and corn flour mixed with water.

Simmer for another 30 minutes or until the stock has reduced down. Drain the carrot and Swede, and mush them well. Spoon-feed the cottage pie filling into two microwaveable dishes then add the carrot mash mixture and season with freshly ground black pepper. Let these cook under the grill for about twenty minutes if you are eating right away, or put them in the fridge for later use, but be sure to cover with a cling film.

21. Asparagus, Ham, And Courgette Baked Frittata

Ingredients

10 chopped asparagus

1 large sliced courgette

80g chopped lean cooked ham

1 teaspoon of dried thyme

4 tablespoons of oat bran

6 eggs

Low fat cooking spray

1 tablespoon of fat-free cream cheese

Salt and pepper to taste

Instructions

Spray the bottom of a non-stick pan with low fat cooking spray. Put the courgette, and fry it gently, while stirring occasionally so that both sides are cooked and browned.

When the courgette starts to brown, add the thyme and asparagus, and simmer for around 10 minutes while adding a little hot water so that the veggies do not burn. Season with salt and pepper once the asparagus begins to soften. Remove from heat and set aside to cool for about 15 minutes.

Pre-heat the oven to 180 degrees C.

Mix the cream cheese, oat bran, and eggs using a fork or a hand whisk in a bowl until a smooth mixture is formed. Dip in the vegetables and ham then mix well.

Pour the egg mixture into a silicone made cake tin. Put in the oven for about thirty minutes to cook until the frittata is done.

You can serve hot or cold.

22. Tandoori chicken

Ingredients

4 tablespoons of fat-free natural yogurt

2 skinless chicken breasts

4 tablespoons of fat-free cream cheese

3 teaspoons of tandoori spice mix

10 cherry tomatoes

10 asparagus tips

Salt, and freshly ground black pepper to season

A bag of mixed leaves salad

Instructions

Make cuts on each of the chicken breasts to make space for the marinade flavors to penetrate, and for stuffing the cream cheese before cooking.

Pour the fat-free yogurt in a bowl, and blend in the tandoori spice mix. Make sure they have properly mixed before you cover with the cling film and refrigerate to marinate for about two hours.

Pre-heat the oven to 180 degrees C.

Remove the chicken from the fridge, and place on a baking tray lined with greaseproof paper. Press in the fat-free cream cheese into the spaces you created in the chicken breasts, and season with the freshly ground black pepper.

Find another baking tray to place the asparagus tips, spray it with low-fat cooking spray, and add a little salt and pepper to the asparagus tips to season.

Place all the trays in the oven for thirty minutes until the meat is done and turns golden brown, and the asparagus tips begin to crisp.

Divide the salad leaves and place them into two plates, add tomatoes, and the asparagus. Add tandoori chicken breast and serve.

23. Curried Cauliflower Soup

Ingredients

1 small roughly chopped cauliflower head

2 finely chopped cloves of garlic

1 chopped small onion

2 teaspoons of curry powder

2 teaspoons of grated fresh ginger

1 teaspoon of ground coriander

1 teaspoon of ground cumin

2 ½ pints of reduced-salt vegetable stock

1 teaspoon of chilli powder

2 herb-flavored oat bran galettes to serve

Low fat cooking spray

Instructions

Prepare the spice sauce by mixing the garlic, spices, and the ginger and 2 tablespoons of water in a small bowl. Mix well until a paste is formed.

Spray the bottom of a tall pan with low fat cooking spray and fry the onions on low heat until they turn translucent.

Add curry paste and cook gently for 1 minute. Add the cauliflower, and cover with the vegetable stock. Simmer gently for about 30 minutes until tender. Remove the pan from heat, and blend everything in a hand-blender.

Serve solo or combine with proteins from oat bran galette flavored with your favorite herbs.

24. Sage And Butternut Squash Soup

Ingredients

A handful of fresh sage leaves

2 small peeled, de-seeded butternut squashes cut into large chunks

2 ½ pints of reduced salt chicken stock

½ onion, chopped

Freshly ground black pepper

Low fat cooking spray

2 herb-flavored oat bran galettes to serve (optional)

Instructions

Pre-heat the oven to 200 degrees Celsius. Line a baking tray with greaseproof paper.

Put the butternut squash in a tray, spread the sage leaves uniformly over the squash, add some freshly ground black pepper and spray with low fat cooking spray.

Slide the tray into the oven to cook for about 40 minutes, or until the sage leaves are crispy and the butternut squash turns tender.

Before the squash is set, find a tall pan and spray the bottom with low fat cooking spray, and fry the onions under medium heat until translucent.

Transfer the sage leaves and the butternut squash into the pan and cover.

Simmer for 15 minutes. Remove the pan from heat then put its contents in a blender and blend until smooth.

Serve on its own or flavor with oat bran galette flavored with your favorite herbs.

25. Red Pepper Fajitas and Chilli Chicken

Ingredients

For the oat bran galette

2 whole eggs

4 tablespoons of 0% fat Greek yogurt

4 tablespoons of oat bran

1 teaspoon of dried thyme

1 finely chopped, green chilli pepper, seeds removed

For the chilli chicken

2 red peppers

2 small chicken breasts

2 teaspoons of hot chilli powder

1 small onion

Low fat cream cheese

A handful of chopped flat leaf parsley to serve

Instructions

Prepare the spicy oat bran galette, and add the thyme and chopped green chili to the batter before cooking. Set aside to cool when ready.

Chop the chicken into chunks, and slice the peppers and onion then mix all of them in a bowl.

Add in the chili powder while stirring to make sure that the peppers, chicken, and the onion are nicely flavored.

Preheat a griddle pan over high heat for about 5 minutes. Place the chicken and vegetables on the griddle pan and cook until the meat turns golden brown.

Divide the oat bran galettes between two plates and uniformly spread with low fat cream cheese.

Top it with the spiced chicken, and add the chopped parsley to garnish. Serve when hot.

26. Nicoise Salad

Ingredients

2 small salad tomatoes, sliced

1 bag of mixed leaves salad

1 large can of tuna in brine (185g)

2 hard-boiled eggs

A handful of green beans, fresh or frozen

1/2 butternut squash (optional)

A drizzle of balsamic vinegar

Optional step for the butternut squash

Pre-heat the oven to 180 degrees C. Skin, then cut the butternut squash into smaller cubes and place on a baking tray lined with greaseproof paper. Spray with low fat cooking spray and cook in the pre-heated oven for some 40 minutes until tender.

Put the green beans in a food steamer and cook as per the manufacturer's instructions. Steaming is highly recommended to ensure that there is minimal loss of vitamins and nutrients. You can also cook in the microwave or boil them in hot water until soft.

Hard-boil the eggs in boiling water for about 10 minutes while you wait for the green beans to cook.

Start preparing the salad when the eggs are set and the green beans have cooled down. First, place the salad on a plate then add the tomatoes, the butternut squash and the green beans.

Divide the eggs into quarter bits, and top them on salad. Place the drained tuna on top then spread with balsamic vinegar.

27. Tomato eggs

Ingredients

4 eggs

Vegetable oil spray

Half a large onion, chopped

3 tablespoons of warm water

400g can of chopped tomatoes

Salt and pepper

A few roughly chopped leaves of fresh basil

Instructions

Spray a non-stick pan with vegetable oil spray then heat it over medium heat and gently fry the onions until translucent.

Add 3 tablespoons of water and tomatoes, and mix well. Let these cook while covered on low heat for 10-15 minutes. Add a little more water if the sauce starts to get too thick and sticky.

Add the basil and stir well to make sure that tomatoes absorb the sweet basil aroma. Break the eggs and pour at the top of the sauce then add salt and pepper to taste and cover again.

You will know if the eggs are ready when the egg whites turn solid while the yolk is still runny.

28. Chicken Greek Salad

Ingredients

1 peeled and diced cucumber

300g of diced cooked chicken

1/2 red pepper, diced

3 diced medium salad tomatoes

1 tablespoon of dried oregano

½ small red onion, finely sliced

Olive oil spray

1 little gem lettuce

Instructions

Mix all the ingredients in a bowl, spray with some olive oil spray and serve.

29. Turkey Mince Mushrooms

Ingredients

800g canned chopped tomatoes

600g turkey mince

½ red onion, chopped

8 chestnut mushrooms, quartered

1 packet of chilli con carne spice mix

1 tablespoon of extra virgin olive oil

1 teaspoon of salt

125ml of boiling water

4 tablespoons of low fat natural yogurt

Instructions

Pre-heat the oven to 180 degrees C.

Mix all the ingredients in a microwaveable casserole dish and cover with the lid.

Slide the dish into the oven for 1 ½ hours to cook until the sauce becomes thick while stirring occasionally like after every thirty minutes so that it does not stick.

Add low fat natural yogurt to each portion.

30. Dukan Cocktail

Ingredients

200g of 0% fat Greek yogurt

150g of cooked cocktail prawns

1 tablespoon of chopped chives

A pinch of paprika

1 tablespoon of Tabasco sauce (optional)

A squeeze of lemon juice

Instructions

Pour the Greek yogurt in a bowl and blend in the chopped chives, lemon juice, Tabasco sauce and paprika. Mix well until all ingredients have blended, and then blend in the prawns until they are fully covered with the sauce.

Sprinkle with paprika and serve when cold.

31. Sea Bass Fillets With Oat Bran Crust

Ingredients

4 tablespoons of oat bran

4 sea bass fillets

A handful of finely chopped fresh flat leaf parsley

2 tablespoons of water

Freshly ground black pepper

The leaves of a few sprigs of fresh thyme

Extra virgin olive oil spray

Instructions

Pre-heat to 180 degrees C under oven grill or grill only if your microwave doesn't have this function.

Place the sea bass fillets without the skin in a greaseproof paper lined with a baking tray.

Prepare the breadcrumbs by mixing the oat bran, herbs and water in a bowl using a fork. The oat bran should absorb the water quickly and take the look of coarse breadcrumbs. Daub a layer of these breadcrumbs on each fillet and spray with low fat extra virgin olive oil spray.

Slide the tray into the oven and cook for about12 minutes, or until the fish has been well cooked. Return the tray to the microwave and place it right under the grill, for another 2 minutes until the breadcrumbs turn brown.

32. Asparagus Soup

Ingredients

A few drops of extra-virgin olive oil

400g of asparagus, roughly chopped

½ large onion, finely chopped

A pinch of nutmeg

500ml of chicken or vegetable stock

Salt and pepper to taste

Instructions

Heat a few tablespoons of extra-virgin olive oil in a non-stick pan and gently fry the onions until they turn translucent.

Add the asparagus and let these cook for a few minutes to let the asparagus absorb the sweet flavors from the onion and oil.

Pour the chicken stock into the pan to cover the asparagus completely. Let these cook until the asparagus is done.

Remove the pan from heat, and add salt and pepper to taste. Blend in with a pinch of nutmeg until smooth.

33. Fennel Gratin

Ingredients

2 tablespoons of low fat cream cheese

2 large fennel bulbs

2 tablespoons of oat bran

Vegetable oil spray

Salt and pepper

Pre-heat the oven to 180degrees C. Slice the fennel into thin slices, and put in a microwaveable dish. Let these cook for about 15 minutes in the oven. When they are set, remove from the microwave, and blend in the cream cheese. Add salt and pepper to season.

Transfer to a microwaveable dish, add the oat bran and spray with vegetable oil spray.
Place in the oven for 30 minutes to cook until the oat bran turns golden brown.

34. Chicken and pepper casserole

Ingredients

A few drops of extra-virgin olive oil

2 large cubed chicken breasts

½ large finely chopped onion

1 yellow sliced pepper

6 thick sliced chestnut mushrooms

2 teaspoons of corn flour

1 red pepper, sliced

300ml of chicken or vegetable stock

A sprig of rosemary

Salt and pepper

Instructions

Pre-heat the oven to 180 degrees.

Add corn flour to the chicken in a bowl to lightly coat the cubes. Place a pan with oil under medium heat and gently fry the chopped onions until translucent.

Add the chicken and leave to cook over low heat until it starts to brown. Add the mushrooms, thyme, and peppers. Simmer for another five minutes.

Add the stock, let it boil and transfer to a casserole dish. Place a lid over the dish, and cook in the microwave for 45 minutes until the chicken becomes tender.

35. Sea Bass Fillets with Oat Bran Crust

Ingredients

4 sea bass fillets

2 tablespoons of water

4 tablespoons of oat bran

The leaves of a few sprigs of fresh thyme

A handful of finely chopped fresh flat leaf parsley

Low fat extra virgin olive oil spray

Freshly ground black pepper

Instructions

Pre heat the oven to180 degrees C.

Place the sea bass fillets in a baking tray lined with greaseproof paper, skin side down.

Blend in the oat bran, herbs and water in a bowl using a fork to prepare the breadcrumbs. The oat bran should soak the water quickly to look like coarse breadcrumbs.

Add a layer of breadcrumbs on each of the fillets, and spray with low fat extra virgin olive oil. This will give the oat bran a nice and crunchy feeling.

Slide the tray into the oven and let the fillets cook for about 12 minutes, or until the fillets are properly done. Grill them for another 2 minutes until the breadcrumbs brown.

Consolidation Phase Recipes

36. Kale and blueberry smoothie

Ingredients

1 tablespoon Almond butter

1 cup of Frozen blueberries

6 ice cubes

A handful of Kales

1 cup of Nonfat Vanilla Greek Yogurt

Instructions

Combine all ingredients in a blender and blend until smooth.

37. Cottage Cheese Jelly

Ingredients

Fat free Cottage cheese (250g)

Boiling water

Jelly lite

Instructions

Dissolve the jelly in a bowl with boiling water then set it aside. Put the cottage cheese in a blender and process until smooth.

Add the cottage cheese to the jelly, and mix until everything combines well. Transfer these into cups or bowls, and refrigerate until properly set.

38. Spaghetti Squash

Ingredients

Spaghetti Squash

Salt and pepper to taste

Instructions

Make some holes in your spaghetti squash by piercing with a knife. The purpose of doing this is to let out steam while cooking.

Slide into the oven for about 4 minutes to cook for every pound.

Leave this to cool once it is done before you continue.

Divide lengthwise to let out the seeds.

Remove the pasta-like strands then add salt, and pepper. You can add your favorite spices.

39. Oat bran granola

Ingredients

2 tablespoons of oat bran

Sugar free syrup

Instructions

Blend in the sugar free syrup and oat bran in a microwavable bowl.

Place in the microwave for one and a half minutes.

Let this cool and then serve with yogurt.

40. Petits Pains D'Avoine

Ingredients

½ teaspoon Baking powder

2 tablespoons of Fat free cottage cheese

2 Eggs

Oat bran

1 cup of Salt fat free yogurt

Instructions

Pre-heat the oven to 200 degrees C.

Mix all the ingredients until smooth.

Pour the mixture into a silicone baking dish then bake for 20-25 minutes before serving.

41. Salmon with ginger

Ingredients

2 Garlic cloves

Ginger to taste

1 Salmon Fillet

2 tablespoons Low sodium Soy sauce

50 ml Teriyaki sauce

Instructions

Preheat the oven to 250 degrees C.

Put the salmon in a silicone baking dish and then add the remaining ingredients.

Seal the foil so that it takes the shape of a parcel while leaving some space inside for air circulation.

Let this bake for fifteen minutes.

42. Turkey Bacon and egg sandwich

Ingredients

2 oat bran galettes + your favorite herbs

2 eggs

8 low-fat turkey bacon rashers

Freshly ground black pepper

A pinch of dried dill

Sweetener to taste

Instructions

Pre-heat the grill to 180 degrees C.

Blend the oat bran, egg, sweetener, and yogurt together until smooth to make your sweet pancake.

Lightly grease a non-stick pan and place it under medium heat until hot. Pour in half of the mixture then add a pinch of your favorite dried herbs and cook the pancake on both sides until golden brown. Put this in a plate and cover to keep warm.

Place the turkey rushers in a tin foil lined baking tray and place under the grill for around 10-15 minutes to cook. Before it is set, poach the eggs using the swirl method, or a poach pod by spraying each pod with cooking spray, and breaking the eggs into the poaching pod; but be careful not to break the yolk. Add a pinch of dried dill then place the pods in a large pan with boiling water then cover and let them cook for about four minutes.

Place the bacon over the oat bran galettes, and top with a poached egg on each. Add freshly ground black pepper to season, and serve.

The Seven Day Meal Plan

Day One

Breakfast

Scrambled Eggs With Smoked Salmon

Beat 2 eggs in a bowl and add a little skim milk. Add chopped smoked salmon then slide in the oven on high for 1 minute. Stir and return to the microwave for some 30 seconds and serve.

Lunch

Ham rolls

Ingredients

175g finely chopped extra-lean ham

225g fat-free quark

Finely chopped chives and marjoram, to taste

4 finely chopped shallots

Tabasco, to taste

Instructions

Blend all ingredients and roll to make small balls.

Dinner

Vietnamese beef

Ingredients

1 tbs oyster sauce

400g sirloin steak, cut into 1cm cubes

3 drops vegetable oil

2 tablespoons soy sauce

Coriander leaves to serve

1 big grated piece ginger

4 crushed garlic cloves

Instructions

Mix the ginger, sauces, beef and a little black pepper. Place in the fridge to marinate for 30 minutes. Cook in a pan until the garlic turns then add in the beef and simmer over high heat for 15 seconds. Sprinkle coriander at the top then serve.

Day Two

Breakfast

200g fat-free yogurt sprinkled with 1 drop of vanilla essence, sweetener and oat bran.

Lunch

Oat bran pancake

Ingredients

1½ tablespoons of oat bran

Dried herbs (optional)

1½ tablespoon fat-free quark

2 eggs, separated

175g smoked salmon, flaked tuna, chicken or ham

Oil, for cooking

Instructions

Blend the oat bran with herbs and a pinch of salt and pepper then add in the fish, meat or chicken and egg yolks. Beat egg whites until stiff peaks form then fold into the oat bran mixture. Pour into a non-stick pan that has been oiled and wiped with kitchen paper and a few drops of oil.

Cook for 2-3 minutes each side.

Dinner

Baked fish with herbs

Ingredients

800g white fish fillets

300g fat-free fromage frais

4 eggs

5 tablespoons chopped herbs

3 drops vegetable oil

Instructions

Preheat oven to 220°C. Add salt to the fish fillets and wrap in greaseproof paper. Place in microwave for 10 minutes then remove and mix the cooked fillets with herbs, eggs, and fromage frais. Pour mixture into a baking dish.

Put this into a bigger dish then fill the bigger dish halfway with cold water and place in the oven for 45 minutes.

Dessert

Lemon cheesecake

Ingredients

4 tablespoons fromage frais

2 eggs

200g cottage cheese

4 tablespoons quark

2 tablespoons corn flour

300g fat-free cream cheese

Grated lemon zest of one lemon

8 tablespoons sweetener

Instructions

Pre-heat oven to 160°C. Mix all ingredients but the corn flour and egg whites and beat until thick and smooth. Beat the egg whites until stiff in another bowl and then add the corn flour.

Pour this into the first bowl. Bake for 40 minutes or until risen and golden brown in a microwaveable dish. Cool, garnish with grated lemon zest and serve.

Day Three

Breakfast

Oat bran porridge

Mix 2 tablespoons of oat bran with some little wheat bran, sweetener and skim milk.

Place in the oven for 2 minutes.

Lunch

Rosemary Beef Burgers (Serves 3)

Ingredients

1 onion, chopped

750g minced beef

2 tablespoons plum sauce

2 garlic cloves, crushed

2 tablespoons finely chopped rosemary

1 tablespoon Worcestershire sauce

1 egg, lightly beaten

1-2 tbs finely chopped basil or mint

Optional Salad to serve

Salt and pepper to taste

Instructions

Mix all ingredients then shape into patties and transfer to the microwave then microwave until golden brown on both sides. Drain on paper towel.

Dinner

Fishcake (serves 1)

Ingredients

6 tablespoons fat-free quark

3 eggs, separated

1 garlic clove, crushed

1 tablespoon corn flour

1 white fish fillet, chopped

Chopped herbs, to taste

3 crabsticks, thinly sliced

Instructions

Beat egg whites until stiff. Blend in the other ingredients and bake at 180°C for 45 minutes.

Dessert

Chocolate Coffee Meringues

Ingredients

2 teaspoons cocoa powder

3 egg whites

2 teaspoons of very strong coffee

6 tbsp of sweetener

Instructions

Preheat oven to 150°C. Beat the egg whites until stiff then blend the cocoa with sweetener and then spread over the egg whites. Add in the coffee and beat for another 30 seconds. Transfer into small mounds on a baking tray and microwave for 25 to 30 minutes.

Day Four

Breakfast

Oat Bran Muffins

Ingredients

8 tablespoons oat bran

4 eggs, separated

½ teaspoon sweetener

4 tablespoons fromage frais

Lemon zest or cinnamon

Instructions

Pre-heat oven to 180°C. Beat egg whites until stiff then blend in the other ingredients. Press in egg whites then transfer into cases and bake for 20-30 minutes.

Lunch

Prawn And Egg Salad (Serves 2)

Ingredients

4 teaspoons cider vinegar

1 teaspoon olive oil

A few sprigs tarragon

600g lettuce

4 eggs

200g cooked and shelled prawns

Instructions

Prepare vinaigrette with vinegar and oil, then season with salt and pepper. Blend tarragon leaves prawns and lettuce in a bowl.

Dip the eggs in boiling water for six minutes until soft then remove shells and serve hot with prawns and dressed lettuce.

Dinner

Salmon Escalopes

Ingredients

2 chopped shallots

4 thick pieces of salmon

6 teaspoons fat-free fromage frais

1 tablespoon mild mustard

Finely chopped dill, to taste

Steamed asparagus (optional)

Instructions

Place salmon in the freezer for a few minutes and then cut it into thin slices. Gently fry these slices in a non-stick pan for 1 minute on both sides then set aside while warm. Cook shallots until brown then add fromage frais and mustard and simmer for 5 minutes. Put the salmon back into the pan and sprinkle dill and season with salt and pepper then cook until set and serve with asparagus.

Dessert

Chocolate Pannacotta

Ingredients

2 egg yolks

2 gelatine leaves

1 tablespoon protein powder

1 tablespoon of cocoa powder

5 tablespoons fat-free fromage frais

100ml skimmed milk

Instructions

Soften the gelatine in a bowl with cold water then combine the cocoa powder, egg yolks, and protein powder in another bowl and set aside. Boil milk in a small saucepan then pour in the egg mixture and stir to mix.

Drain excess water from the gelatine and blend into the hot mixture until completely dissolved. Let this cool, before adding the fromage frais.

Day Five

Breakfast

Skim Milk And Muesli

Ingredients

1 egg

6 tablespoons oat bran

Almond essence

1 tablespoon liquid sweetener

Instructions

Preheat oven to 160°C. Blend all ingredients and place on baking-paper-lined tray. Bake for 30 minutes. Wait until cool then crumble. Preserve in an airtight container.

Lunch

Salmon Pancakes

Ingredients

60g fat-free quark

300g fat-free fromage frais

4 slices smoked salmon

1 small jar salmon roe

2 oat bran pancakes

Instructions

Blend the roe, quark and fromage frais in a bowl and season. Split this among pancakes and top with salmon.

Dinner

Chicken Kebabs

Ingredients

1 peeled garlic clove

1 onion, peeled

2 tablespoons lemon juice

20g grated ginger

½ tablespoons ground coriander

100g of fat-free plain yogurt

1 teaspoon garam masala

½ tablespoon ground cumin

800g chunked chicken breasts

2 tablespoons finely chopped coriander

Tzatziki, to serve

Instructions

Purée garlic and onion in a blender. Blend in lemon juice, coriander, ginger, spices, and yogurt. Add marinade to the chicken then chill for 2 hours.

Preheat the grill on high then place chicken on skewers and place on the grill. Leave to cook for 8-10 minutes and then serve with fat-free tzatziki.

Dessert

Orange Yogurt Cake

Ingredients

150g fat-free natural yogurt

3 eggs

1 teaspoon orange extract

½ teaspoon artificial sweetener

2 teaspoons yeast

4 tablespoons corn flour

3 drops of vegetable oil

Instructions

Preheat the oven to 180°C. Blend eggs with yogurt, and then add orange extract, sweetener, yeast, and corn flour. Pour into a cake tin and bake for 45 minutes.

Day Six

Breakfast

Scrambled eggs and smoked salmon

Lunch

Asian soup

3 liters fat-free chicken broth

1 yellow onion

2 knobs fresh ginger

Chinese black rice vinegar

2 cloves star anise

¼ cup soy sauce

Snack

Mediterranean chicken drumsticks

90ml prepared mustard

30 ml fresh rosemary

15 ml fresh cracked black peppercorns

30ml fresh thyme

15ml salt

2 lbs chicken drumsticks

Dinner

Nicoise Salad And Lemon Mustard Sauce

Nicoise salad

1 can tuna packed in water or juice

3 tablespoons of capers

Fresh dill to garnish

1 quartered hard-boiled egg

4 scallions, chopped

Lemon-Dijon Dressing

Lemon Mustard Sauce

3 tablespoons fat-free yogurt

3 tablespoons Dijon mustard

1 mashed garlic clove

Day Seven

Breakfast

½ cup of berries

Soft boiled eggs with meaty crisps

Lunch

Oat bran pancake

Smoked salmon appetizer

Snack

10 almonds

Dinner

Roast chicken with some vegetables. Ensure that the chicken has no skin.

Conclusion

Thank you again for purchasing this book!

I hope this book was able to help you know how you can lose weight with the Dukan Diet as well as simple recipes that you can try at home to lose weight.

I wish you the best of luck with your health and weight loss goals!

Thank you again for purchasing this book!

Sara Banks

Disclaimer

Please remember that anything discussed here does not constitute medical advice and cannot substitute for appropriate medical care.

71499418R00040

Made in the USA
San Bernardino, CA
16 March 2018